Precious Memories on Life's Journey

Precious Memories on Life's Journey

MARGARET E. PECKFORD
(NEE KING)

iUniverse, Inc.
Bloomington

Precious Memories on Life's Journey

iUniverse books may be ordered through booksellers or by contacting:

iUniverse
1663 Liberty Drive
Bloomington, IN 47403
www.iuniverse.com
1-800-Authors (1-800-288-4677)

ISBN: 978-1-4620-1743-0 (sc)
ISBN: 978-1-4620-1744-7 (ebk)

Printed in the United States of America

iUniverse rev. date: 05/05/2011

CONTENTS

ABOUT THE AUTHOR

Hi! My name is Margaret Elsie Peckford (nee king). I was born in the old King family home in Victoria Cove, Newfoundland, to Annie May and Esau King on August 30th 1944. I was the fourth child in a family of eight and I spent my childhood years growing and learning how to be the best that I could be to my fellowman. I was married at twenty to a wonderful man who after forty seven years is still by my side and we had four beautiful children together.

I remember well the poems and short stories that I wrote as a child and believed then that someday I would realize my dream of writing a book. Now happily retired after dabbling in a few career opportunities; my favourite been a Registered Massage Therapist; I now enjoy my time writing and reading as well as singing in a church and community choir. I also serve in other church activities such as Secretary of vestry, chair-person of Altar Guild and a member of the Anglican Church Woman.

I am truly blessed with precious children and grandchildren with whom I love to spend time as much as possible. I equally enjoy spending quality time with my husband in and around the little town of Appleton, Newfoundland where we live. I also enjoy travelling on cruises and staying in beautiful resorts in different parts of the world.

I have had six poems and three short stories published in the Poetry Institute of Canada Anthology of Verse.

God is good. May love, light and laughter fill your hearts today and always.

ACKNOWLEDGEMENTS

Thank you to all my family and friends who shared some of their stories with me. Thank you to my friend Gary John who has kindly written the Preface for this book.

To my brother Roy King; I am eternally grateful to you for editing my book. To everyone who helped in any way with this book I thank you. A very special thank you to my tireless assistant my Lord and Saviour Jesus Christ who has inspired me and given me strength and courage to continue when times have been difficult in my life. To all those who believe that love is the answer, let your little light shine.

DEDICATION

I dedicate this book to my husband Laurence who has supported me from day one.

This book is also dedicated to my wonderful children Angela, Paula, Trevor and Evan, as well as my precious grandchildren Eric Nicole, Daniela, Lauren, Brandon, Kailey and Tailer, and great-grandchildren Darion, Reis and Damion who are and always will be the joy of my life. Thank you for letting me grow with you along the journey.

PREFACE

What a wonderful read, that took me back to a simpler way of life from the past. Even though I did not grow up in the same place of Newfoundland as Margaret did, the echoes of a lot of our childhoods are similar indeed, and brought out through these pages.

How many of us can relate to a ``Mr. Hopkins,`` the old school, school teacher who was a beacon of light to all of his fortunate pupils. A person who really fits the cliché of `` they broke the mold when he was born.``

I felt a warm glow as I read the stories of love for her Mother and Father, her husband and children. Margaret`s poems prose, and stories are all told from one place and that is from her heart.

From childhood trials in the hospital, to wonderful relatives who inspired her, to the tragedy of a loss of her own child, all these poems are both inspiring and poignant.

Her sense of God is present in all of her writings, from her very earliest times. The serenity with her beliefs is embedded throughout all of her words.

I entreat you to take an hour of your busy life, find the nearest rocking chair, have a glass of wine in one hand and this volume in the other, and re-live your own past, whilst reading Margaret`s wonderful heartfelt words.

Blessing to my friend Margaret.

Gary John

A LITTLE PILGRIM'S JOURNEY

I heard you calling from the mountain,
Thundering through the valleys;
Humbly I listen, awakening to the sounds of the universe;
Conscious of the connection of body, mind and soul;
I journey through the valleys and peaks,
Sometimes silent, sometimes deep emotions in my soul;
My spirit broken, lonely, afraid, ultimately shattered,
I journey far into the night.

Darkness fills the night, animals and birds return to their
nests,
Except for the Owl whose spirit is awake;
Forlorn and weary, I tuck my head into my chest.
I cry out in anguish, I pray to my creator, Dear God,
Expel the darkness and bring me to the light.
Morning breaks, I lift my broken body, my spirit refreshed.
I see a rainbow beyond and hope fills my soul.

With open eyes I see creativity and beauty all around;
Brilliant colours and a voice gently saying, "I will not
abandon you;
Look beyond, my little pilgrim, child of the universe,
Your journey has just begun; you are a special, unique,
valiant being
Traveling onward, even in your weakest moment"
Thank you, creator God, a guardian angel journeys with me,
Forever in body, mind, and soul, connecting you and me.

A journey of a thousand miles begins with a single step. (author unknown)

A TEAR DROP FELL

A tear drop fell,
As I stood in my own silence;
A cloudless sky;
The sun scorching the farmer's fields,
As oxen strained under the plough;
Fragments of debris lay in the streets.
The wind blowing sand through the alleys,
And 'round the cold square cement buildings.
Tattered garments hung
From balcony windows;
Half open doors swung back and forth.
Men, women, and children
Lined the walkways for handouts,
Each person received their rash-ions.
Workers looked burdened from a hard day's work,
But smiling with a $10 monthly wage in their hand;
The once magnificent stone buildings
Of the 1500-1900 hundreds,
Now torn, faded, and left to ruin.
Devastation all around;
Cries from a child;
A man praying to a marble statue,
Of a woman with a baby at her breast;
My prayer today was for my arms to be
Big enough to enfold them all to my breast;
Yes I stood in silence in a crowd,
Praying;
With teardrops falling

Go to him each morning for strength to meet the day have faith in God—He is your
friend(author unknown)

A TINY RED ROSE

I mixed the soil in my own backyard,
With sunshine from above;
I planted the seed in my garden,
And I watered it with love.
It was just a tiny seed,
Each night the bud did close.
I watched it daily as it grew.
It soon became a rose.

I dreamed I was fashioned like that rose,
Was beautiful, graceful, and loved;
I heard my own heart beating,
From the soft breezes up above,
My body was clothed in petals,
So soft was I to touch.
My love was burning from within,
Just waiting seemed too much.

I need so much to give you dear,
That perfect shapely rose.
But thorns have scared them deeply,
And many a rose has closed.
But today I give you one red rose,
All my love is wrapped within.
Accept it darling, it's from my heart,
To you, my love, my friend.

The fragrance always remains in the hand that gives the Rose.(author unknown)

AUNT HARRIET

My eyes filled with tears that day;
Her heartaches I tried to share,
But no one but the Lord above,
Knows what a cross she bore.
A face that was lined with wrinkles;
The silver in her hair;
A picture of a woman,
With love beyond compare.

Mother, Sister, Aunt, and Friend,
On the pages of Gods roll;
Also Great, Great, Great, Grandmother,
With the Lord you will abide

What a wonder to behold.
Your hands so small and shaky now;
A heart that is old and worn;
A lap that made the world seem small,
With your arms around us thrown

You gently rocked us in your chair,
And hymns we sweetly sang.
Your voice rang out like angels,
As you held us by each hand;
There will be a star in your crown forever,
To replace the thorns in your side;
There will be sunshine in the valley,
Yes she is ready for the roll call,
Because she has lived a life worthwhile;
Forgiveness she has asked for,
And God has granted with a smile.
Dear Jesus will be waiting,
When she reaches Heavens door;
She will cross the banks of Jordan,
Where sorrows will be no more

Death ends a life but not a relationship.(author unknown)

4

AUNTIES GIFT OF LOVE

You could tell by her stature that she might have been a fairly tall lady in her younger years, but now she was a little bent and crippled. She looked smart in her pretty green bonnet that matched the car coat she was wearing. On her arm she carried an old, worn, but neat basket with a few items wrapped in bright tissue paper

In front of her at the little county post office, stood a tired looking, middle aged man, who wore a torn jacket, and had a sad look on his face. She tugged at his coat sleeve a couple of times, and with the kindest look on her face, asked him if he would choose a gift from her basket. Almost in disbelief he turned to stare at this little lady with the thickest eye glasses that he had ever seen. He hesitated for a moment, but then he chooses a gift. The lady saw that his face took on a big rainbow smile that lit up the little room. Through his tears of joy he thanked her and left the post office saying "My Sarah will love this". It was a beautifully designed brush and comb set.

I couldn't take my eyes off this lady, and we were no sooner out the door when she said to me, "My dear I can't do this now like I used to, I'm not all that strong" Then taking my hand in hers, she gently but firmly gripped it. With a smile she said, "My name is Molly, but everyone around here calls me Auntie."

As we walked along I told her my name. She told me that when she was very young she had the measles, and since there weren't many Doctors around, she didn't get proper care, and the illness left her with respiratory problems. She said, "Through the years it caused emphysema which I have dealt with all my life." Taking a couple quick breaths, she said, "Now if I get to coughing real bad just give me a few hard pats on the back and I will be fine again."

5

I thought; we need more people like Aunt Molly. She had a hump on her back, crippled legs and from what I could see sparse teeth, but a heart as big as the moon and she carried it on her sleeve.

As we came to a turn in the road, she said, "This is where I live," pointing to a quaint little dwelling, at the end of a narrow path, just off the main road. Until now I really hadn't said much, but to my surprise I asked her if she needed help getting up the steps, "Sure thing" she said, so I took her by the arm and up the old, worn steps we went.

You could see the joy on Molly's face when she was greeted by her grey and white cat, which she called Dusty. With a jolly big laugh she said, "He dusts for me you know." Then sadness crossed her face and she said, "He is all I have now that my husband died; me and Dusty and my daily basket of gifts to those less fortunate than myself." I thought, what a lady, gathering dust maybe, but gathering flowers for the masters bouquet was more like it.

She talked some more, then she looked at me, with the most beautiful smile and said, "My Mom always said if you couldn't say something good about someone don't say anything at all, and you're going to be just like my Mom." "What did you say your name was my dear?" I thought patience man patience, and I gave her my biggest and most special smile and said, "Good Night Auntie, Good Night."

As I walked away I noticed her long fingers. A piano player I bet in her day. I bet she could still play a few tunes. What a lady, I thought again, small and frail in stature, but like a mountain erupting with love.

It's nice to be important but it's more important to be nice. (unknown author)

BLACK ISLAND IN THE SEA

By Margaret Peckford

We went out to Black Island,
One lovely summer's day,
With Mary, Glenn and Dylan,
With these friends we're going to stay.
Marjorie, she's Glenn and Danny's mother,
And she's only eighty four.
She told us many funny stories
And anecdotes galore

We stayed in this awesome cabin,
Built with tender love and care,
By the hands of Glenn and Danny,
Their skill shows everywhere.
Mary and Carolann added their special touch,
With pictures and decor so neat,
Add Dylan, Danielle and Tyler,
And it made this awesome cabin complete.

Now, to get out to Black Island,
You have to cross the water deep.
Sometimes the hills are oh so high,
I could close my eyes and weep.
Now, when you come to the end of the boat ride,
The island beauty shows its worth.
With the sun rays reflecting on the water:
The moon shining down on the land of their birth

Now, no one has to rough it,
Because this cabin is complete;
A large kitchen, electric lights and showers;
A toilet and a sink;
The beds are built into the wall:
Don't forget your king sized sheets.

Margaret E. Peckford

There's a wood stove in the corner,
That throws off quite a bit of heat.

Now, we're here for thanksgiving weekend:
We have so much to be thankful for:
The salt fish and the porridge,
The turkey and fresh vegetables galore
Today the men are turring,
So the ladies they will cook.
We'll knit and write and walk the trail,

Then sit and chat or read a book.
You are a very special family,
Yes you're such a happy crowd.
If your ancestors could see you now,
They would be very proud.
Today we go back to point of bay:
We hope the seas are not too rough,
For the women got nothing to hold on to,
Because the men got no hair on their scruff

Laurence and I will never forget,
The kindness that you've shown
Thank you from the bottom of our hearts,
And yes, you're welcome in our home.
We had an awesome weekend,
With friends that have great worth.
We are privileged to have enjoyed,
A little heaven on this earth;

In the trees and flowers of the field, in creatures great and small we trace the watchful care of
him who planned and made them all,(author unknown)

CHRISTMAS MEMORIES

Christmas memories in Newfoundland; I know my pen won't fail me now that I need to express, with reverence, a subject so special to me. I hope to stir the hearts of many as they reflect, with me, on some of the memories of the past. I grew up in a little out-port in Newfoundland during the forties and fifties with a Mom, Dad, four brothers, and three sisters. Grandpa and Grandma also shared our five bedroom two story home.

I was most fortunate to be part of this three generation family. Each of us, from age one to eighty, made memories and shared special occasions together, one such time being the twelve days of Christmas. The innocence of youth and the wisdom of the aged gave us all the opportunity to learn the real meaning and spirit of Christmas. Please join me now as I journey back in time.

It is Christmas Eve, and a green fir tree with the ice glitter still clinging to its branches sits on the porch. In the kitchen the clinking of pots and pans attests to Mom and Dad preparing tomorrow's feast. The roosters who proudly strutted their stuff just this morning, now lies freshly plucked and ready for the seasoned stuffing. Vegetables and figgy puddings have been made and set aside in bowls.

Grandma sits in her flour barrel rocking chair, wearing a long dark dress with a white lace collar. A shawl is draped over her bent shoulders and a large white, starched apron almost reaches the hem of her dress. She wears her hair parted in the middle and pulled to the back of her head in a bun. Hair pins are attached to keep it tidy. Melvina, Elizabeth is a distinguished looking lady, but even so, she always keeps a watchful eye on the children.

It is time for the children to get their baths, a couple at a time are put into a large washing tub and it is pulled over by the stove for warmth. Grandma makes sure that their ears are cleaned and that their necks are at least a little red from the scrubbing. Then after a hearty supper, they don their pyjamas or night gowns, which were carefully made by Mom out of colourful flannelette, especially for Christmas Eve. Prayers are said, and after hugs and kisses Mom or Dad tucks them in bed for the night. That old familiar song, warning all children to watch out and not cry, rings out in spurts and starts, and is heard all through the house.

The household is now buzzing with activity. The Christmas tree is brought in and set up. As tradition goes, the little children will not see the tree until morning. The older children with Mom and Dad are putting up decorations, hanging bells from the beams and criss-crossing garland, made from crepe paper, and stringing it from one corner of the room to the other. Streamers made from popcorn, coloured paper rings, and the ornaments that the children made and covered with silver, gold, and red candy wrappers, are hung on the tree. A star made from cardboard and covered in shiny foil is humbly placed on top of the tree. Among the decorations they find a box of bulbs that are wrapped in tissue paper. Their eyes light up when they hang them from the branches, as they are so delicate in texture and show different colours in three dimensions. Then they all stand in awe, as they look upon the decorated tree.

It is now time to begin stuffing woollen socks, everyone has one, but they are all shapes and sizes. The smaller gifts are now tied to the tree branches; the bigger ones will be placed around the tree later. This is also the time for the singing of carols, shaking heartily the hand of aunts, uncles and cousins who drop by sharing gifts, and to wish everyone a Merry Christmas. Everyone is thankful for another year even though it was oft times marred with sickness and death. But now the family is ready for sleep, because early tomorrow morning the pitter-patter of little feet and the echoes of laughter will ring through this out-port home.

Christmas morning; a soft blanket of snow covers the earth as if to blot out the impurities of the past year. The children scramble out of bed and shout out Merry Christmas, as they race down the stairs to see if Santa Claus came.

Tradition reigned in our home. By now, Mom and Dad have the porridge pot on the stove and the smell of toasted bread teases the nostrils. The younger children are looking at the tree for the first time. Their eyes sparkle and are bulging out of their heads; they are amazed at the beauty of the tree and the gifts around it. They wonder aloud if it's real or if it's magic, because it had appeared so quickly. The children then get their stuffed stockings and empty the contents. Between squeals of delight they bite into a five point apple, take out an orange, some grapes and a few hard shelled nuts. Although there are no fancy nutcrackers, a hammer and a piece of wood are placed on the floor for them to use.

Everyone is anxious to get to the stripping of the tree, and see what's inside the beautiful wrapped gifts. But tradition still stands. Tummies filled, Dad now reads from the Bible. It is a true test of endurance as the younger children try not to wiggle and giggle, as they kneel in a row by the day bed, for family prayers.

At last, prayers are over, and the names are called. Each child squeals with happiness as he or she opens a gift. The girls receive tiny bottles of Ben-Her and Jasmine perfume wrapped in a delicate white, embroidered handkerchief. Times are good when each girl gets a doll. One excited little girl gets a doll with a stuffed straw body, earthen head, hands and feet. The doll is dressed in rich red fabric, and its face is painted to perfection, with rosy cheeks and sky blue eyes, that look almost real.

One niece spends a lot of time with Aunt Emily and Uncle Fred; therefore, at Christmas she received a white wash-stand with a flattering pattern made, with love, by Uncle Fred's very own hands. After fifty-five years it is still one of her most treasured possessions, and stands in a place of honour, in her Newfoundland home. On top of the wash-stand sits a wash-bowl, pitcher and a soap dish. In the cupboard, underneath, there is a chamber pot, ready for an emergency.

Now for the boys, they are thrilled with their five blade pocket knives. Now they can make whistle pipes out of alders, like Dad taught them. They think that, maybe, they can impress the girls with them. Then they see the larger packages, wrapped in red paper. With shaking hands they tear them open to find skates. Wow! Another dream came true. The excitement mounts as another of the boys sees a red and white Coaster (sled) behind the tree.

The children have been saving pennies all year and have carefully chosen gifts for Mom, Dad, Grandpa and Grandma. The women are delighted with a pretty pink box of dusting powder, with its very own puff, and a tiny bottle of gardenia perfume. The men are pleased with their new shaving brushes and mugs, complete with razor blades. Everyone gets homemade mitts, scarves and socks, and if Mom wasn't too crippled with arthritis, everyone got a knitted sweater to keep them warm and brave the winter storms. The whole family now share hugs and kisses and thank everyone for the gifts.

With a gleam in her eye, Mom scurries everyone to get dressed in their best winter clothes and dash for a seat in the sleigh. Dad snaps the reins, and the jingle of old Dan's harness bells ring out loud and clear in the morning air. The sleigh runners sliding over crystalline snow squeak loudly as they make their way to the little village church. Grandpa helped build this church, and he is proud to be with his family, celebrating the birth of Jesus. Everyone's spirit is soaring, and they are letting their little light shine, as they reminisce with family and friends. The message of Peace on earth, Goodwill to men, is evident in this quaint house of God.

The cold, frosty air has blossomed into roses on the children's cheeks. They walk in the door of the church and their eyes light up like magic when they spy the green boughs with red bows that decorate each pillar, as they walk toward the altar. Candles are glowing on the altar, and the scent of myrrh reminds them of what they learned in Sunday school about one of the gifts brought to Jesus, by the Magi. They gaze in wonder at baby Jesus lying in a manger. Then the choir of voices, young and old sing, "Hark the Herald Angels Sing, Glory to the New Born King."

Then it is home for Christmas dinner. A dozen or more family members gather around a large table, with chairs that have an exquisite hand carved design, evidence of Grandpa's skilled workmanship. Inside the table is a long bench, which can seat five or six children. Blessing is given and then all eyes are on the big, juicy, roasted roosters. Some want a leg and others a wing. Somehow, Mom always finds a way to keep all her children happy. They all feast on the colourful vegetables. The stuffing, the figgy pudding, and the delicious gravy all tickle their tonsils. While eating dinner, they reminisce about last Christmas or catch up on some happenings that are going on in the family. Like who lost a tooth, when would they wear their new dress, and when was Grandma Squires coming to visit?

After eating such a hearty meal and giving thanks they roll away from the table feeling like the stuffed rooster they had just eaten. After clean up, Mom and Dad get a little rest while the children play together with the gifts that they received.

Holiday festivities continue for the twelve days of Christmas, or until old Christmas Day, which is January sixth of the New Year. One of the special occasions is the Christmas Concert. All the school children and teachers take part in dressing up and acting out dialogues, singing, reciting recitations and short plays. One angelic little girl in the family dresses up like a Christmas tree and recites a monologue.

On Boxing Day, the ancient Roman custom of mummers begins. Young and old dress up in old gowns, fisherman's oilskins, or any crazy outfit they can find. They top this off with hats and ugly masks. Pillows are also stuffed in appropriate places to create disguise. They go from home to home, knocking on doors, and in a cracked voice ask "Will you let the mummers in?" No one is turned away and the fun begins. One of the mummers takes an accordion from under his oversize gown and the sound of music fills the home, as he plays a jig called "Turkey in the straw." Everyone grabs a partner, and all from Grandma to the children are out stomping out a jig in fine style, even with their rubber boots on.

Now it's time to pass the bottle. Homemade blueberry and dogberry wine is a special treat for the adults. The children are pleased with lemon crystals or cherry and orange syrup, a true Newfoundland tradition. The fruit cake, that has been seasoning since early fall, is brought out. What a delicious taste and the fruity smell makes ones mouth water. Hot peppermint is also served to anyone with a tummy ache, even if it is only from laughing. If a mummers name is guessed, he is relieved to remove his mask for awhile, and get to wipe the sweat from his brow.

New Years Eve is also very special in Newfoundland. Church service is attended by almost everyone. At midnight the church bell rings out, guns are fired and can be heard all over the little community. Young and old are wished a very happy and prosperous New Year. Lots of New Year's resolutions are made, and young lovers make promises to each other. On beautiful moonlit nights folks take long walks in the freshly fallen snow and make a wish upon a falling star. The night sky is spectacular, the air is frosty, and the New Year is welcomed, in true Newfoundland spirit, by singing course after course of "Auld Lang Syne."

It's Old Christmas Day. The tree and all the decorations are down for another year. The Children are back to school; Mom is back to her knitting and Dad is cutting wood for next winter. Two thousand years ago a saviour was born in a stable in Bethlehem to show us that light can shine in darkness and that love can live in our hearts forever.

Grandma, Grandpa, Mom and Dad have gone to their heavenly home. All eight children are living in several areas of Canada and are all doing well. At our family reunions there is lots of reminiscing about the good old days of Christmas. Fifty-five years later memories still flood my heart, especially as I write of the happiness that I experienced in our Newfoundland home, especially during the twelve days of Christmas. It was a precious journey back in time. I hope you enjoyed it too.

Count your many blessings and you will soon lose count. Author unknown

FORGET-ME-NOT

Forget me not my special friends,
As the flowers bloom again this spring;
My thoughts return to those special spots,
To the old church lane and the forget-me-not's;

The flowers grew each side of the lane.
In fields of blue each year the same.
I remember picking them from a tiny tot
To ask family and friends to forget-me-not;

Each year in my own little garden patch,
The flowers bloom for the sun to catch.
While they grow in the sunshine my memories flow
To the old church lane from long ago;

When I look at the flowers they mean so much,
That I pick a few just to feel their touch;
Then I offer a prayer to God for the sun and the rain,
That the flowers will grow and bring sweet fragrance
again;

Over sixty years have passed but I feel just the same,
As when I picked those flowers in the old church lane:
The colour and sweet smell bring memories that don't
stop,
For family and friends and the sweet forget-me-not;

All creation is an outstretched finger towards God. (author unknown)

GOD'S PRECIOUS GIFT—A SON

In loving memory of Trevor Laurence Peckford
Who died from SIDS February 17, 1967

It's still hard to talk about, or ask God the reason why,
My baby boy was taken, I remember with a sigh,
How I fed and rocked him close that night,
Not knowing that by morning he'd be taken from my
sight.

I cried out in anguish, "Please Lord don't let him be
dead."
I cradled him in my arms and moaned, as I lifted him
from his bed.
Not a sound came from him, no smile upon his face.
It tore the heart right out of me, "Please God, grant me
grace."

No words can tell you how I felt, or how deep I hurt
within.
The guilt, the anger, the disbelief, this can't have
happened to him.
The pain it tore my heart and soul, as sadness filled the
morn.
It was ten to eight in the morning, the same time that
he was born.

I lost part of me that day, with no chance to say
goodbye.
Now over forty years have passed, and I still ask God
the reason why.
He was three months and twenty-four days, when God
he called him home.
God loaned me a precious gift, then he needed an angel
for his throne.

I had three other precious children, and a husband that
I loved.
They filled my heart with many joys, and I thank the
Lord above.
But there is no one that can take his place, the vacant
spot is there.
Each time the family gathers, I see that empty chair.

I know he's gone to be with Jesus, around Gods
heavenly throne.
God loved Trevor very much, that's why he called him
home.
Time has helped heal my broken heart, yet still the hurt
remains.
The day will come when I'll be called and I'll see him
once again.

Death leaves a heartache no one can heal, Love leaves a memory no one can steal. Author
unknown

GRANDDADS CLOCK

When I just a little girl,
About eight or nine years old,
I remember Granddad as he rocked in his chair,
And the funny stories that he told;
The clock chimed once.

Granddad sure could chat a bit,
And any subject was fair game,
Religion, law or politics,
The sunshine or the rain;
The clock chimed twice.

He would chat and chat and chat some more,
Then he would get up off his chair,
The door would be swung open now,
'Cause I am leaving now he would say my dear;
The clock chimed thrice.

His great big boots made three of mine,
And he stood over six feet tall,
He chopped the wood and built the barn,
And filled the water barrel that stood against the wall;
The clock chimed four.

Now Granddad was a God fearing man,
No one took him for a fool,
He went to church on Sunday,
And tried to live by the golden rule;
The clock chimed five.

He prayed and buried and baptized,
And the lessons he did read,
From the good book each Sunday morn,
The gospels and the creed;
The clock chimed six.

He helped the neighbours mow the grass,
And cleaned their snow filled walks,

He picked up the children after school,
And listened while they talked;
The clock chimed sevenWe lived up around the cove,
Granddad said that it was at least a mile,
And many a stormy morning,
The King children had to toil;
The clock chimed eight.

Our little feet would soon get cold,
And our fingers almost freeze,
But soon we'd be to granddads house,
That was just beyond the trees;
The clock chimed nine.

Granddads home was big and warm,
Because he was up at break of dawn,
He'd call us in to warm our hands,
And then he'd sing our favourite song;
The clock chimed ten.

Abide with me his voice rang out,
Bless be the tie that binds,
Don't cry my child be brave and strong,
And then we'd hear the chimes;
The clock chimed eleven.

I can picture him now when he stood in the pulpit,
A mighty but gentle man,
His voice could make the rafters ring,
But he could kiss a child's hurt hand;
The clock chimed twelve.

Then one day Granddad wasn't there anymore,
To warm our hands and feet,
But he'll sing with the angels in heaven I'm sure;
Like the clock made its circle, his life is complete.

A parent's life is a child's guidebook. Author unknown

I PONDER

I Ponder! Did Jesus look like you and me?
When Joseph cradled him on his knee;
Was Jesus dressed in ribbons and bows?
No, Jesus was wrapped in swaddling clothes.

I Ponder! When Jesus cried did Mary sing him to sleep?
When he was aroused by the cattle and sheep;
Yes and angels sang and helped him to rest;
When he cuddled close to Mary's breast.

I Ponder! Did Jesus have a Christmas tree?
Gifts tied to the branches for all to see.
No! In Bethlehem there was hunger and strife;
Joseph and Mary could only give birth.

I Ponder! When the Wise-men came from country far,
To worship the king, they followed a star.
They each had a gift but it was not fur,
They gave him gold, frankincense, and myrrh.

I Ponder! The Shepherds too, they followed the star,
Right up to the stable with the door ajar.
They found Jesus in a manger, so humble and meek,
Then fell down to worship at Jesus feet.

I Ponder! Did Jesus have a load of toys?
Just like our little girls and boys.
No, he brought us life by way of the cross,
And peace on earth, so we wouldn't be lost.

I Ponder! Will our gifts be simple and sweet?
Will we lay all our treasures at Jesus feet?
No, most of our gifts will be pricey and big;
Too big to lay down by Jesus' head.

I Ponder! Will you come to the altar this Christmas
morn?
Will you shout Alleluia that Jesus is born?
Will you remember that Jesus in a manger did lay?
And still gives us blessings this Christmas day.

I Ponder! Do you think when Jesus looks below?
He still sees strife like long ago.
But he walks with us, if there's room in our hearts;
He'll be our Saviour and from us never part.

JOURNEY OF AN AGED MIND

"Hello Aunt Harriet" I said, as I pulled up a chair beside her bed and gave her a hug and a kiss. She said hello, but I could tell by her expression that she wasn't sure who I was. It had been two years since I had been home from Alberta to visit her. But, before I had the chance to tell her who I was, she said, "Oh, I know who you be, you're Margie, my Brother Esau's daughter." She took both my hands in her worn and wrinkled ones and tears streamed down her face, she was laughing and crying at the same time, she was so happy to see me.

I don't know what I expected to see when I walked into the Lakeside home that February day in nineteen ninety-three, but I will be forever thankful that I took the time to go there. As I first gazed at my Aunt, I saw a lonely, old woman with wrinkled hands and face, with shoulders bent forward on her shrunken body, and legs that were no longer strong enough to carry her around, without the help of a walker.

Then, I looked again and I saw the most beautiful woman, shining with love, joy and peace in her heart. It filled me with strength and courage. I had the overwhelming desire to take her in my arms and cradle her, and tell her that everything was going to be all right. In that moment I remembered the words of the old song, "Rocking Alone in an Old Rocking Chair, I Saw an Old Lady with Silvery Hair." But to me, that day, my Aunt looked like an angel rocking in her chair.

With that beautiful smile of hers, she looked up at me and said, "The Blessed Lord will soon take me now; I've told him that I'm ready, but I'm worried about my son Nelson, he'll be all alone when I go, because his Dad passed on a few years ago." She trembled and cried again, and told me that she worked hard in her day and had loved and lost a lot of loved ones along the way.

Aunt Harriet was always special to me. The wisdom that she passed on to me on her visits each summer stayed with me my whole life. She would tell me stories, and was always so happy to sleep in the same bedroom that she slept in as a child. She would touch the clock in the kitchen, look with pride at the pictures on the wall, tell me about how she churned butter in the old butter churn, and spun wool on the big spinning wheel. She said, "If those walls could talk they would have many a story to tell." Then she told me how she caught the barnatickles, and played dolly house out on the bar by the big white rock.

By now, I had spent several days doing regular visits with her, and had truly awakened her senses especially about her youth. She said, "I worked from sun up till sun down my dear. My dad owned his own schooner and spent a lot of time fishing on the Labrador. All hands had to help poor mother; she was an angel you know. So, I helped with spreading the fish, turning the hay, setting the vegetables, and shovelling snow in the winter. I also milked the cows and fed the goats and sheep and when sheep-shearing time came I would help catch them in the lane between Esau's and Fred's."

She also told me about going to school and church. "We had to learn everything by heart, the Lord's Prayer, Creed, Catechism, and even the Collects. Not at all like today my dear. I can still recite some today". Then she rattled off a poem titled "From the Cradle to the Grave." She spoke about my Dad and Mom, Esau and Annie, "Your Dad was a funny guy; always had a story to tell, and your Mom, she was a very special lady, I loved her so much." With tears in her eyes she said, "Your Dad died at age sixty-one and your Mom at sixty-seven, and here I am ninety-four and still living. What does all this mean?"

I reminded her that God always has a reason for his timing, and that I felt honoured and blessed to be able to sit and share with her the stories from her past. I reminded her that in nineteen eighty-nine she was awarded a certificate from the Guinness Book of Records for being the youngest Great, Great, Great, Grandmother in the world. That was a tribute to a very special Lady. I also told her that I couldn't imagine my childhood without an Aunt Harriet.

With tears streaming down my face, I enfolded her in my arms and told her how precious she was to me, and how thankful to God I was to have journeyed this special time with her.

It's not the years in your life but the life in your years that count. (author unknown)

LEGACY FOR BECKY

What can I leave you?
Money I have none;
No riches at my feet.
No satin robes or precious jewels,
Can this poor man bequeath?
So short our time,
But much I have to give.
Our memories, richer than gold;
These I leave.

You can keep that little grin,
The smile, the laugh that warmed my heart;
The star we borrowed from the universe;
The wish we made and one single teardrop.
I'll grace you,
With one early morning dawn, one moon,
One star-filled night;
My strength I'll give you when you are weak.
One dream, one kiss, my love to keep.
This to you I do bequeath.

Success is not the key to Happiness. Happiness is the key to success. Author unknown

LIVING WITH DEPRESSION, THROUGH CHRIST

In the United States and Canada, millions of people are suffering from depression. Not so long ago "feeling down" was thought to be merely an unfortunate state of mind, for which the affected person was largely responsible. Today, however, the medical world sees depression for what it really is, a disease, which is devastating but treatable.

Depression just doesn't pick a person to attack like one would choose someone to read or sing. It can strike young, old, rich, poor, black or white. Some of the symptoms of depression are similar, but the effects of these symptoms are not always the same for each individual. This often makes it difficult for the medical profession to match the correct treatment with the person.

Some of the symptoms of this disease are poor concentration, weeping for no known reason, insomnia, unfounded fear, and unusual thoughts such as dwelling on suicide, hearing voices, feeling unworthy and seeing things that are not there. There are also physical changes such as weight loss or gain, nausea, little or no interest in sexual activity or to the other extreme. Headaches occur, as well as the fearful feeling of not wanting to be seen outside your own little corner. Another symptom is avoiding phone calls and visitors at all costs.

The depressed person can be very low in spirit and vitality; wishing to be alone all the time. Then the mood could swing to the other end of the spectrum, and the person become high with uncontrolled behaviour, needing lots of company. Both scenarios can bring on uncontrollable spurts of crying and hurtful feelings that last for an undetermined period.

I have had my own experience as a depressed person. But I am living proof that one can be depressed through your whole life and with help still maintain a fairly active family, community, and spiritual life. From a spiritual and Christian viewpoint, I would like to tell you about some of my experiences, and explore some healthy avenues that helped me, which I feel will help others live with this debilitating disease.

One of my many counsellors, with empathy said, "You are a sick person, who is sometimes well." Yes I thought, he really hit the mark. As far back as I can remember I felt different. My depression began at an early age. I always felt that I was slow to learn school activities; slow to develop compared to other teens; thus I remember being called names and pushed around a lot by my school class mates. I felt the odd one out and that I just didn't fit in with the "In crowd".

I didn't feel worthy, even when something good happened to me. I remember the time that the school voted for the most popular girl and boy in Girl Guides and Boy Scouts to present a Bible to the church. Peter Record was the boy and I was the girl. I was so excited until I heard some of my class mates say that it shouldn't have been me that was chosen. The day of the presentation should have been one of the best days of my life, instead it was terrible. I stood there at the altar feeling unworthy, unloved and actually ugly in my Girl Guide uniform. As tears streamed down my face, that day, I looked out in the pews and saw Mom and Dad with a big encouraging smile, and I knew in my heart that they loved me and were very proud of me. That's what got me through, and also because they always taught me that Jesus loved me, no matter what people said.

My teen years were a struggle. I told myself that everyone would be better off without me. I used to cry a lot and I felt like I was a burden. I always felt like I'd failed in everything I tried to do, and I couldn't get past that. Then, I felt that I had let Mom and Dad down. They worked so hard for all of us. There were eight of us and Mom was sick a lot and Dad had to be away from home to go to work. I missed him so much, and it was difficult for me to understand that he had to be away to earn money to support us.

Through those early years I suffered from depression not knowing what it was. I did most of the things that teenagers do. I was in the Brownies and Girl Guides, and I took part in school concerts. I dated several boys, and of course, I thought that I was in love with most of them. I went to times, as we called them then, and danced the night away. I baby-sat to get a little pocket money. Then when I was eighteen all that changed; I went to Lewisporte to work.

While in Lewisporte I met, fell in love, and married a wonderful man who still stands by me today after forty-seven years of marriage. We had four beautiful children two girls and two boys. Our first son died at three months and twenty-four days, of crib death, now known as SIDS. This is a parent's worst nightmare, and I was no exception. Two weeks before our son was born my dad died of cancer. I couldn't go to see him because I was pregnant, but still three months later he died anyway. I was angry with God, and every fibre of my being was shattered. Within days I sank as low as I could go, yet I still managed to look after our two girls and my husband. It was at that time that I received my first medical treatment for depression. I was very scared and again feeling unworthy and guilty that I was seeking professional treatment. In the small community where I lived being depressed was bad enough, but to be seeing a psychiatrist really labelled me.

Today, as I recall my depressed state, I will try to put into words what my feelings were when I was experiencing some of my worse moments. I felt like I was in a deep, dark pit, with walls so slippery that there was no way for me to get out. No escape, no refuge, only the ugliness of feeling unworthy. Even in my bed, which I felt was my only sanctuary, I would pull the blankets over my head and close my eyes; even the light was distasteful to me. I didn't want to get up; I didn't want to see anyone or go anywhere. I was trapped in utter darkness. It is difficult to describe what ones emotions and actions are to anyone who has never experienced depression. At one time I would make excuses for my thoughts and actions, but not anymore, because I now know that in this desperate, depressed state, one has no control over them.

After several different kinds of treatment were tried, that were unsuccessful, it was decided that I would be admitted to the hospital for Electric Shock treatment. That's another story in itself that I won't go into. But after the shock treatment, months and months of psychiatric sessions followed daily, until I began to learn how to deal with my feelings of unworthiness, guilt, and unwanted thoughts, that were taking over my life. This seemed to be the last ditch effort to heal from this dark place, and replace it with love, and hope for the future.

Some of you are probably saying, she should be thinking about what she has; her loving husband and beautiful children. Well, it was then that I did think of them. What was I doing to them, why can't I be different? I prayed like I never prayed before, to get well and to be a better mom, wife, and daughter, to the ones I deeply loved. At my Mom and Dad's knee I was taught the Lord's Prayer and that Jesus loved me and that he would always be there for me. If I ever needed Him, I needed Him now, so I prayed in a still small voice. Yea though I walk through the valley of the shadow of death I will fear no evil: for thou art with me: thy rod and staff comfort me.

My most vivid memory of the shadow of death was when I was in the hospital on a stretcher, in a row of twenty to be taken for Shock treatment. I felt like I was being taken as a lamb to the slaughter. Then I remembered the passage of scripture in Genesis, where God tested Abraham with his son Isaac. God saved Isaac, so I prayed that he would save me to.

Through the years I have been on several different kinds of medication. Antidepressant drugs, tranquilizers, and stimulants, all of them powerful and complex chemicals. Some years ago, I was finally diagnosed with By-Polar depression. Now, I am very thankful to be only on one pill a day for depression. I will always have to struggle with this disease, but with God's help, and the love and support of my family, I am able to maintain a really good quality of life.

This only scratches the surface of what I've dealt with, but this is not only about me, it's a story to tell others; that you can live a productive life being a depressed person. Those of you, who suffer from depression or have someone who does, please don't blame them. Actually don't blame anyone; it is a DISEASE that affects millions.

Never avoid medical help, and find compatible groups to help you through the difficult times. My prayer for you would be for you to have an understanding husband and children to stand by you. The light at the end of the tunnel seems far off sometimes, but believe me there are lots of good times to treasure, so cherish them all, the births, school days, birthdays, graduations, weddings, and anniversaries. Love and support from family and friends will always help you through. Finally, love through Christ. Have faith and believe in the Lord Jesus Christ, and know that he will always be there for you. He is the wind beneath your wings.

"You may not always win the battle but you will win the war."

The rough roads of life are often the ones that bring us closer to Christ. (author unknown)

I sought to hear the voice of God and climbed the highest steeple but God declared "Go down again" I dwell among the people. Author unknown

LOOK CLOSER

If you see your friend in sadness,
And you can even see the awful strain.
Please don't think that they don't want to,
Hear your voice call out their name.

Maybe their day just didn't go right.
They might choose to wear a mask.
Try to help them forget their sadness,
Just by taking time to ask.

Why not be a little patient,
And chat with them for just a minute.
Next week their story might be different,
Because you took the time to be part of it.

So remember when you see their face,
Don't judge them by what you see.
Deep within is all their power,
That's the true face they can be.

Keep your words soft in case you have to eat them.(author unknown)

MILLY'S MENAGERIE

There were dolls, hundreds of dolls, in all shapes and sizes, and in a kaleidoscope of colours, in Milly's home and garage. Milly smiled as she invited my Aunt Jean and me into her world of magic. Milly was ninety-one years young, and her glowing face expressed the excitement of the four year old that she was when she received her first doll. Milly sipped her green tea, which she said helped to keep her young, and then she asked us to join her as we looked and talked about her collection.

"This was my first doll; it was given to me by my Auntie." She pointed to an elegantly dressed doll that was standing in one of her many glass cabinets. Standing next to her was a doll that was two hundred years old, dressed in posh ivory silk and lace. We asked about this doll but Milly only knew that it was from Ireland and was a gift to her.

While we were looking and talking about the dolls, Milly began to tell us about her life on the farm, where she and her husband raised their family. She told us that her husband had his first of three heart attacks before he was forty. So, besides all the hard work on the farm "I got myself a part-time job and a hobby. That was almost sixty years ago, and this is what I have today," she said, with a nod of her head. With another brilliant smile she took us to see her two sailor dolls. "That's the first two dolls that I bought after I took the part-time job at Tom Boy's grocery store to help support my hobby."

Some of her dolls were gifts from family and friends, and from all over the world. For some of them she filled out Royal Crown Soap and Campbell's Soup coupons. She then reached out her hand and switched a button and Elvis Presley in his white attire twisted, shook, and sang in his smooth romantic voice.

A couple of steps further, we stared in disbelief at the Beatles, all of them with perfect hair and style, with instruments in hand, as if ready to perform. Apparently there was a story to tell about purchasing the

Beatles. Milly found herself in an older part of the city of Edmonton, in an under-ground, cellar-like store, somewhere, where she had never been before. With a slight toss of her head, she pointed to the Beatles and activated them so they sang in all their glory.

Shirley Temple, from the thirties, sat next to a telegraph operator equipped with glasses and ear-phones. Standing with his horse, and dressed in his Red Serge was a R.C.M.P. officer, representing the Musical Ride and Canada, back in eighteen seventy three. At that time they were known as the North West Mounted Police (NWMP). There were dolls from Alaska, Lapland, Greece, Spain, and Cuba. There were pram dolls from England, called Bisque. Also in the line up were two African American dolls, from New Orleans, that were only two inches tall and one hundred years old.

At the touch of a button her frog dolls danced to a lively tune. Then we saw Popeye the Sailor Man with his spinach and his sweetie Olive Oil, sitting lovingly together. We saw dolls made from rope, from Bermuda. Dolls made from waste paper from Mexico. There were T. Eaton dolls from Canada crowded next to Gerber baby dolls all ready for their dinner. Little Miss Muffet was sitting with dolls that could laugh, cry, burp, suck on soothers and pucker up. Excitement showed on her face as she showed us her Bobby Cop doll from England and her set of Beauty and the Beast dolls.

My Aunt and I complemented Milly on her glowing face, her beautiful complexion with no wrinkles; she said. "I never wore make-up in my whole life; I spent that extra time caring for my dolls."

On our way down memory lane we came to her Barbie doll collection; they range from baby to adult, gypsy to queen. She had Barbie in her wedding gown, and she even had a pregnant Barbie. "My mom would come back from the dead if she knew I had this one," she said in a whisper, removing the clothes from the very pregnant doll. Milly's face was priceless, actually with the glow of a "pregnant Momma." We mustn t forget her partner, the handsome Ken doll, in his unique attire, standing by her side.

Milly was beaming and having a grand time showing us part of her life, as she put it, through the image and beauty of her dolls. Next, she showed us her flapper dolls from back in the twenties. There were kitchen witches, and Colonel Sanders standing proud, showing his broad grin.

Campbell Soup dolls lined her kitchen cupboards, along with, the friendly Pillsbury Dough Boy.

Then we were led to the garage. Now, in most garages you would likely see a car and other odds and ends, but not Milly's. Her garage was lined with wall to wall carpet and, of course, wall to wall dolls. In a cradle with pillows and matching blankets were twins, dressed only in diapers. "Check inside the diaper and see what gender they are," she urged. Sure enough there was a boy and a girl, with all the trimmings, even to the umbilical cord. Shelves lined the whole of the garage. Sitting on one shelf were her Kewpie dolls, a unique collection, ranging from two inches in length to thirteen inches. On another shelf, sitting in the corner, was the famous Dennis the Menace, from the early sitcom, sharing his mischievous grin.

Milly was the proud owner of a King George doll from nineteen hundred and two. Catherine the Great stood proud and tall in a rich organza, red fabric dress flowing to the floor. Beside her was another special doll, dressed from Ireland. We also saw dolls from Paris, China, Spain, and Holland. There were dolls with long hair, short hair, curly hair, and some with no hair at all. A few more steps along, sitting on the shelf, was her three-in-one, Little Red Riding Hood, of course, the little girl, Grandma, and the big, bad wolf. Beside them were her old man and old woman with their arms around each other, and a loving smile on their faces. She said "They are enjoying their twilight years, my dear."

Milly then showed us a Cinderella doll. "This is the last doll that my husband gave me before he died." She wound up a spring in the back of the doll and it played a touching love song. It brought tears to her eyes and ours as well. But nothing kept Milly down for long. "Come over here and see the one and only Lucille Ball, as always she's looking smart and chipper." Standing beside her in stately fashion was the whole collection of Ann of Green Gables, from Prince Edward Island.

Now, an hour had gone by, so I asked Milly if she wanted a break, after all she is ninety one years old, but no, she still wants to go on. Next we went to see the older dolls, some with cracked earthen faces; they were dressed in pretty pinafores with bonnets to match. Raggedy Ann and Andy graced the next shelf, looking adorable. Daisy and Donald Duck, Mickey Mouse, Lucy and Linus, and the Smurfs were sitting or standing and looked so life like that they could have been going to a party at Disney World.

There were dolls in baskets, on tables, sitting, standing, in cribs, highchairs, rocking chairs, lying on pillows, on lifebuoy soap boxes, and wrapped in blankets of every color, inside Milly's home and garage. The dolls are made from different materials; some were made from rubber, porcelain, china, plastic, rope, wool, and one from rock. Some are stuffed with straw, wool, cotton, and some with synthetic materials, from all over the world.

Milly told us that her friends and family often make new outfits for some of them, and "If I have more than one alike, I donate one to the senior club for their sale." Another couple of steps and we came face to face with the Butler, he had a wink in his eye, but was ready to attend to our needs.

"Who do we have over here?" asked my Aunt. Milly said, "Oh, that's my Scottish lad. Do you know what he wears under his kilt?" Then quick as a wink, she whipped up his kilt to reveal her Scottish lad in full bloom. Laughter filled the little garage as we chuckled, and admired Milly's sense of humour. Yes she even had "THE GREAT ONE, WAYNE GRETZKY" in his hockey attire. In a small wooden box, on a corner shelf, she showed us a natural Japanese doll with six different wigs that were very bright and colourful. This Japanese doll had been dressed by true Geisha girls.

"Now you look up here," Milly said. What should we see but a large, life-like Brian Mulroney doll, hanging on a short rope? "Yes my dear, I keep him hung from the ceiling." Her face was beaming with laughter, yet with gentleness. Milly's presence itself brightened our day as we continued our walk with her down memory lane.

"Thank you for coming," Milly said. "Many memories have flooded my heart today as I talked about my dolls and things about my life; you have awakened my senses." I then asked Milly what doll she would like to receive next, and in a blink of an eye she said, "Chretien my dear, Chretien, and I'd hang him up with Mulroney, I should say that they would get along together just fine."

What a lady, what an afternoon. Aunt Jean and I will be talking and dreaming about these six hundred plus dolls for a long time to come. Milly's Menagerie was a sight to behold, an honour and a tribute to this special ninety-one year old lady, and an inspiration to everyone who has the opportunity to enjoy life to the fullest, in whatever they choose to do. Last, but not least, Milly's dolls range in price from one dollar to five hundred dollars, but to Milly they are priceless, and the light in her eyes tell us so.

Milly has since gone to her eternal rest and she donated all her dolls to the Westlock
Museum in Alberta. Thank you Milly and God's Peace be with you.

May the hinges of friendship never rust nor, the wings of love never lose a feather. (author unknown)

MY CHRISTMAS

By Nicole Hutchings

Finally school is out 'cause Christmas time is here.
Present shopping for your family and friends who are so dear.
Waking up to your sister singing carols by your door,
Makes you want to cuddle up and fall asleep some more.
Hot chocolate by the fire and candy canes galore,
Ornaments and greeting cards are all over the floor.
Christmas morning has come at last; you can feel it in the air.
Christmas trees with lots of presents all to give and share.
Wrapping paper and boxes all over the floor,
Oh, the anxiety of wanting to open more.
Clothes, cameras, video games and N64,
Games, watches, money and there still is more.
Relations gather to give thanks for the day,
While all the younger children go outside to play.
For the rest of the day light fills the air,
'Cause me with a camera, everyone beware.
It took an hour to eat our dinner, but an hour well spent,
For after that hour to the dishes it meant.
The smell of cookies all through the house,
Cousins eating them up, leaving not one for a mouse.
The day has come to an end but don't you dare fear,
For this episode will continue this very next year.

Every child has a gift some children unwrap their gifts earlier than others. (author unknown)

MY CREDIT UP YONDER

I wonder, what have I accomplished, here on this earth?
There have been a lot of years since the day of my birth.
Now that I have more time to just sit and ponder,
Yes! I wonder, what of my credit up yonder?

I have helped the elderly, the sick and the poor,
With family and friends to achieve a good score;
But I get no credit for good deeds alone,
Like the woman in the Bible, who will cast the first stone?

No, I can't swipe a card, when I reach Heaven's gate,
Or peek at my record to see how I rate.
My account may not balance; I may be overdrawn,
So what of my credit when things are done wrong?

Sometimes I feel that I may need one more round
Before I would warrant a star in my crown;
Yes! How much time do I have to sit and ponder?
Before that great roll call is heard up yonder?

I know that my days are numbered on this earth,
And I count my blessings since the day of my birth.
I believe that Jesus is my Saviour, Lord and Friend,
And if I ask Him humbly, He will forgive me my sin.

There is no extra time to rewrite my script,
I trust I was forgiven each time I slipped.
My eyes will be open as he raises the curtain,
For I'll see by his face what God knows for certain.

The evening of a well spent life brings its lamp with it. author unknown

MY LONG AWAITED CLOTHES LINE

It's been twenty years since I had a clothes line, to my
husband I did say.
I'c like to have one like my friend, who lives across the way.
So off he went and bought a pole, a steel one tall and round.
He dug a hole and set the pole deep into the ground.

I was a happy washer woman and the day it looked so fine.
My basket full of laundry I would hang out on the line.
I was singing gospel music as I hung out my white sheets,
And all the other garments I hung them oh so neat.

A gentle wind was blowing; there was not a cloud in sight.
The sun was shining brightly, a good day I have no doubt.
My white sheets they were flowing like the wings of a dove.
I knew my prayer was answered by the good Lord up above.

About a couple of hours later the wind in Eastern came.
And as the dark clouds gathered it sent down a shower of rain.
To and from the line I went my patience growing thin.
My drawers they now were off the line and going for a spin.

Cut the kitchen door I ran 'cause my clothes were flying high.
The clothes pins they had sprung apart before my very eye.
Now get this off the line I said before my nerves do crack.
Holy smoke! What's on my sheets, the crow had done a crap.

This is it I said to myself as I brought the last garment in,
And threw the sheets back in the wash to do all over again;
Then out came the sun and the gentle breeze right before my
very eyes.
So I hung the sheets back on the line and watched them fall
and rise.

If you don't have wrinkles you haven't laughed enough. Author unknown

37

MY SPIRIT SOARS

My spirit soars because,
You are the eagle flying high,
The wind that makes my wings to fly,
You are the sun up in the sky,
The light that shines as I pass by,
You are the moon that lights the night,
The dreams I dream that I hold tight.

My spirit soars because,
You are the stars of the universe,
The star-dust on my heart that burst,
You are the rainbow in the sky,
The chirping of the birds that fly,
You are the knock upon my door,
The smile on your face I'm waiting for.

My spirit soars because,
You are the rain that waters the earth,
The trickling spring that gives new birth,
You are the mountain, oh, so high,
The hugs I need to get me by,
You are the breath which I caress,
The completeness of my happiness.

I know not what the future holds but I know who holds the future. Author unknown.

NATURE

By Kailey Peckford

I glance outside my open window,
I feel the wind gently blow,
I see bright green trees,
And a few bumble bees.
The bright blue sky has few planes;
It looks as if it never rains.
But all these things that are small,
They add up to it all.
They add up to Nature!

Never be afraid to try something new remember amateurs built the Ark professionals built the Titanic.

SHADOW RIVER

Swallows hovering over the river,
Taking flight;
Driftwood hanging over the banks,
Partly submerged in the river;
Willows blowing in the wind,
On a June summer's day;
A beaver splashed its tail,
And disappeared into the water;
Fireflies fluttering above,
Sparkling with color;
Rapids bursting with glee;
Sapphire sky and,
Trees casting shadows in the water,
On a June summer's day;
Owls sleeping;
Sandbars emerging,
Fashioned by the current;
Bulrushes thriving,
Breathing in the muddy depth;
Young ducklings swimming,
In single file,
Making ripples on the water,
On a June summer's day.

The best things in life aren't things. Author unknown

THE KING FAMILY HOME

In the eighteen hundreds, our family home was built by our Grandfather, Alfred John King. It was two stories high with a steeply peaked roof. What was called a back kitchen was built on, and was used more than any other room in the house. That was the room where all the cooking, knitting, and sewing were done. That's where yarns were told, a child's skinned knees fixed up and a lot of tears kissed away. The inside part, was a special room, where a radio was set up; the one with the big battery attached. That's where Dad would listen to the news, and of course Uncle Mose, the story about Pigeon Inlet. The children also used this room for our Sunday morning service, when it was too stormy to walk down around the cove to church.

Upstairs, there were four bedrooms, a boy's room, a girl's room, a Mom and Dad's room, and the other room was for whomever there were more of at the time, girls or boys. There was a closet at the top of the stairs and a door leading to the attic. The attic was off limits to the children, but that didn't often stop the older ones. When we were playing hide and seek they would hide up there to scare us.

At the bottom of the stairs there was a little hallway, which had more doors in it. One door led to a room that was called a sitting room. It had a little stove in it and was used on special occasions. For a few years it was turned into a bedroom for Grandfather and Grandmother, until they passed on. The front door had beautiful, coloured glass in it. Wide timbers spanned the ceilings, and strong posts and frames divided each room, that made up the King family home.

I remember a story told to me by my mom about Grandma King. Grandma was a very staunch Anglican and faithful in the words of scripture. The Bible was the book of Knowledge and Gods word and anything inside these pages were to her, life itself. She had what she called the SAVIOUR'S LETTER, and had it tucked safely inside her Bible.

She read her Bible every day, but when things would get a little tougher, she would always read the Saviour's letter and believe in it very strongly. This one particular time there was a forest fire raging towards Victoria Cove. While everyone rushed around, Grandma clutched the letter to her heart and prayed and prayed. After many hours of watching in fear, the wind changed and sent the fire toward the ocean, with only a couple of miles between the fire and our home. Many thanks went up to God that night, and a stronger belief than ever in the Saviour's Letter.

Dad was a hard working, honest man, not very tall in stature but big in heart. He tried to bring up all his children by the golden rule. Dad was also a very witty man, a good story teller and could play one hundreds and twenty's with the best of them. He taught us how to play crib as well as crazy eights. At night, he helped us with our home work, whenever he could, by the light of the kerosene lamp. Dad only had grade six, but since he was an avid reader, his education went far beyond his school days. He would read the weather glass and give us the forecast for a few days in advance. He would say "Now, Annie my dear, be prepared for a blizzard because the glass is down to twenty nine. The wind will be in Eastern, and there will be lots of snow." Also in the winter time he would say to us in the morning, "Now, you had better stay at school this evening until I come and get you, because by three o'clock it will be blowing and snowing." Sure enough about two o'clock the wind would be up, and snow drifting around the school. Soon, Dad would be there on old Dan, our horse and sleigh and our teacher Mr. Marcus Hopkins, would say, "Ok, all you children from up around the cove can leave now." We'd all pile on the sleigh and laugh and giggle all the way home.

Dad sawed, chopped, and brought home the fire wood every year. He planted a garden, and filled the cellar with vegetables every fall. When Dad was home, he was always up early and would have the wood stove going to have the house warmed up for the rest of the family. In those days there were no electric heaters to keep us warm, and many a morning our pee would be frozen in the chamber pot. Even the canvas on the floors sometimes curled up from the cold. But a pan of eggs and a pot of Porridge would be on the stove, and Mom and Dad would say "Now eat your breakfast and warm your innards, before you leave this house."

Now, I give Dad all the credit that he's due, and that's a lot, because he worked in all wind and weathers to provide for his family and as you will see through this story that he did many other things. But then there's Mom, the backbone of the family. Mom knit socks and mitts and sweaters. She turned her coats inside out and made coats for us to wear. She wiped our snotty noses, bandaged our scraped knees, and mended our broken hearts. She scrubbed our clothes on the scrubbing board and hung them out in the frosty air, and when she brought them in most times they could still stand alone, they were so frozen. She'd get them dried over the stove or wherever there was a place to hang them. Then with two or three flat irons that she heated on the stove she would iron the white shirts that she had starched. One of our brothers, Mark, was a server on the Altar, so his shirts had to be white, starched, and spiffy.

Mom cooked big scoffs most every day. One day there would be salt beef and doughboys, another day fish and bruise and scrunchions. Another good meal would be a large pot of baked beans with homemade bread, which she made at least every second day. We would also have toutons from the bread dough, which were delicious with black strap molasses and butter. Mom made soups of all kinds; she could put a delicious taste on whatever she cooked. Fresh pork, chicken, and lamb was prepared and cooked in their season, all topped of course, with fresh vegetables from the garden. Mom helped us with our homework, taught us our prayers and made sure we knew the Collects for Sunday school. She kept us on track with our Brownie and Girl Guide uniforms and helped us earn our badges.

Mom and Dad had a big family; there were eight of us in all. I'm sure if the walls could have talked they would have had many a story to tell. Unfortunately, our home burnt to the ground in nineteen eighty one, so what memories we have is tucked in our hearts.

Well, I could probably tell a few little stories. Archie and Roy were the two oldest, and it seems like they were ready to leave home before us girls got to know them much. But I do have one vivid memory of Archie. He loved to tease us girls, and one such time would be when we had our yearly vaccination, our arms would be really sore and Archie would shake our hand and ask how we were doing today. He would especially get Gloria because she would pretend that it didn't hurt and he would keep doing it. I also remember how he could step dance, and we would love to go to the Orange Men's time, so that we could watch him. One night at the orange Men's meeting they were trying to decide what to serve for the meal and Archie suggested Fluffs. He truly was a funny guy, and lots of fun to be around. By the time we were in our teens he had left for

Ottawa to find employment; we were all sad to see him go and as they say the rest is history.

Roy was our musical guy; he played the guitar for hours, and filled the house with songs like "This Old House and Your Cheating Heart." Roy taught school, at Davidsville for a year and came home on weekends. In the wintertime he would walk across the bay on snowshoes. We would watch from the window until we could see him coming around Tippy's Point and then we'd know that he was all right. Then one Sunday morning when the steamer, the Bonavista, came into the cove, Mr. Roy Record took him out in his freighter. He was off to the Army to do training. Another sad time for all of us, as it was a long time before we saw either of them again.

Next were the girls, three in a row. Roxanna was the oldest and the leader of the pack. She had black hair that was straight as a whip. Being the first girl, Mom and Dad were pretty proud. She had pretty flannel dresses and home knit stockings and as soon as she was big enough she had new "lumps" for her feet, which she displayed quite proudly. As the years went by she readily passed on her wisdom to the rest of us, and changed her name from Roxanna to Roxy. Now, I came next, and I was the girl with the round face and chubby cheeks. Mom's friend and nursemaid Nellie used to twist up my hair in brown paper. After a few hours she would take out the papers and my hair would be all curls. Another one of my Mom's friends and nursemaid spoke to me just the other day about how she used to call me Marnie moo. Of course, my name was Margaret, but most times I was called by pet names, Margie or Marnie moo. Later I wore my hair long and had pig tails, that hung down to my butt.

Gloria Beatrice, here she comes! Ready to show the world that she's special. Roxanna and I passed her down some of our hand me downs, and believe me they didn't last Gloria very long. Mom used to say she'd tear up the world in an hour if it was made of material. Gloria could take her part with the best of them, and sometimes took my part as well, when we would get into a tiff at school.

Roxanna, Gloria, and I were best buddies most of the time, we laughed, talked, and played hopscotch and see-sawed and walked to the ice-cream parlour on long summer evenings, each with our five cent piece. We were very proud of our yellow taffeta dresses that mom made for us. We walked to school together, and enjoyed the cocoa malt at the Sunday school picnics.

Then along came another boy. Now, Mark was like a play toy to us girls. When he got old enough we dragged him around with us when we played dolly house out on the bar. He was a cute little thing, with a grin that charmed us and our friends. No one wanted to sleep with him because he rocked back and forth all night long. We were all scared the day he got on a ice pan and floated out the bay. We were all playing copy pans in the beach when he went out too far. Someone went out in a boat and brought him in and he zapped up the attention that he got from everyone then, keeping of course, that special grin. All of us girls looked out for him at school. Mark was a staunch server in the church, under the direction of Rev. Joseph Taylor. The summer of nineteen sixty-six, he went to Ontario to find employment, like his two older brothers.

Enid was the next girl to enter the family and the baby girl of the family. Enid Elizabeth caught the attention of everyone who saw her with her long blond curly hair and big blue eyes. She was daddy;s girl alright I remember him wrapping her up in a big pink blanket and carrying her up to bed each night to tuck her in.

Seven years went by and another baby arrived. A big surprise for everyone, the King family was supposed to be complete; little did we know that the cream of the crop was making his entrance into this family, and that he would bring much laughter, some tears, and many more memories to this family. Lorne was his name, and from the time he started walking at eight months there was someone chasing him, to keep him out of trouble. By now, I was sixteen and wanted to go down the road in the evening to be with my friends. Mom wasn't feeling so well some days and Marnie, as Lorne called me, had to stay home and help Mom with him. He was cute as a button all right because he would pretend that he was asleep in his crib, and then when I would get to the top of the stairs he would cry out to me again. Some nights I didn't get out at all, but because he was my precious baby brother, he couldn't do anything wrong in my eyes. One of the most dramatic things that happened to him was to fall into a large flour barrel. Mom was right there, of course, and when she pulled him out all he needed was a bit of water and he would have looked like the Pillsbury Dough-Boy.

There were twenty two years difference between the oldest and the youngest of the King family. By the time the youngest was born the older ones were away at work. It was not until the summer of nineteen sixty-six, the year that Dad was sick, that we were all home together. Even our cousin, Walter King, was home from Scotland to visit Dad. Although everyone shared a lot of old memories, and recalled events of our childhood, that summer, it was overshadowed by Dad's illness. Dad was diagnosed with cancer of the larynx around Christmas time in nineteen sixty-four. He went through lots of tests, treatments, and surgery, which resulted in losing his speech. Although he was only sixty-one years old and a strong man in his faith, the harshness of cancer finally took him on November ninth, nineteen sixty-six.

Like most families we didn't go through our growing up years without trials and tribulations. There were times when Dad and Mom struggled to make ends meet. Times of grief when loved ones passed on to their eternal rest. Certainly, there were times when us children squabbled and tested one another, and also tested Mom and Dad. I'm sure there were also times when Mom and Dad were tested themselves, and probably wanted to throw in the towel, but somehow they made it through, always showing us children the lighter side of things and making it right for all of us. We have so much to be thankful for, to have grown up in such a large family, with a special Mom and Dad to teach and guide us. We may not have had what some would call the finer things in life, but to us we had it all. We had food on our table, clothes on our backs and lots of love for everyone. We had a kind, loving, and caring Mom and Dad who gave us their all. What more could we ask for? Mom went to her eternal rest at a very early age as well, she was only sixty-seven, and although, she too was strong in her faith, she was weary, and tired and ready to go home.

I have only set your ears burning by touching on a few of my memories. I hope in reading this all of you brothers and sisters will think of other pleasant memories that happened while growing up in the King Family Home, and find comfort in knowing that no matter where we are or where we go, our ties began in the King Family Home. I also hope that any other relatives and friends that come upon these words may enjoy a brief glimpse of what it was like to grow up in this two story house on Tippy's Point.

Bless the food upon those dishes as Jesus blessed the little fishes and like the sugar in our tea may our hearts be stirred by thee. Amen. Author unknown.

WHO, WHAT, WHEN, WHERE, AND WHY

Who will we trust all through our life?
Who will we depend on in our daily strife?
Who will we pray to both night and day?
Who will carry our burdens and cast them away?
Who will it be?

What will be our cross as we tarry?
What will be our portion to carry?
What will we do if we give up the fight?
What will help us to keep our cross light?
What will it be?

When will morning sunrise open the sky?
When will the noon breezes be blowing high?
When will evening shadows suddenly fall?
When will the night bring darkness to all?
When will it be?

Where will we be when the hours have passed?
Where will we be when the weeks go so fast?
Where will we be when the months go so slow?
Where will we be when the years they just flow?
Where will we be?

Why will we hope that we haven't done wrong?
Why will we want to blow our own horn?
Why will we pray for all things to pass?
Why will we know that it's God's love that will last?
Why do we ask?

Fishers of men, you catch them God will clean them, author unknown

A TRIBUTE TO THE MAN OF THE YEAR MR. MARCUS HOPKINS

None of your shenanigans now! Get your heads into those books because you'll be getting a test next week. Review everything from Chapter 10-15. That is only one of the many phrases that we heard from Mr. Hopkins. He was a man of his word. Besides being a husband and father, he was the principal and teacher of the Victoria Cove School. He was the superintendent of Sunday school, Lay reader in the Anglican Church; a member of the Orangeman's Lodge and proudly led all of the parades. He was also the man who threw the candy the farthest at our school picnics.

He was a born leader although he didn't profess to be one. His actions, posture and quick step reflected his quiet self assurance and set an example for everyone. He had enormous knowledge and was proud to teach the golden rules of everyday life to all who would listen.

Of course I can only tell you my childhood memories of this man but I'm proud to say that they are all precious and have stayed with me through the years. One of my special memories is of when I would get to the school on a cold or wet day; Mr. Hopkins would have a roaring fire in the pot belly stove and I would stand there and get warm and a little dryer before class began.

Picture in your mind our little two room school with a porch at the entrance to each classroom. Boys and girls cloak rooms were on either side of each entrance. There was small office in the center accessible from each classroom to accommodate two teachers. At the back of the school were a stage and another room. That room was used as a dressing room when preparations were being made for the concerts and plays that took place every year at the school.

Out back was the coal shed where many a mystery was left unsolved or so we thought. I think with the keen ears and eyes of Mr. Hopkins not much got pass him. The boys and girls privy's were out in front of the school and many a young man's eyes wandered to his favourite girl as she strolled to and from the privy and vice versa. The girls were probably worst than the boys. To complete our school system there was the Parish hall where a third teacher held school for grades one to three.

Mr. Hopkins always opened our school day with prayer and being on time was a must. Roll was called and you were marked present or absent and account kept through the school year. In those days most of us young ones only knew about Victoria Cove, the little place where we grew up; so school and church were very important to us. We had to be at least a teenager to be able to go to Rogers Cove, Wings Point and Cla`kes head unless our parents were with us. The likelihood of that happening would be for a Christmas Concert.

Christmas Concerts was one of the many things that Mr. Hopkins worked very hard at. Each year as sure as the snow fell all students would be staying behind after school to practice for our concert. He would make sure that each of us got a part whether it was a poem, a song, a part in a skit or dialogue as we called it. He gave us the opportunity to gain our confidence to be able to stand on stage for the first time in public and say our bit. He was an inspiration to all who knew him.

In our small communities everyone knew everyone else anc. visiting was done by walking from home to home. Like everyone else Mr. Hopkins walked everywhere except in the winter when he could use the horse and sleigh. Sometimes darkness fell before he got home for supper, however when important matters had to be discussed there was no alternative. Most importantly at the end of the day as they'd say it was done with a handshake and a smile.

I can see him now as he called the roll in the morning, in his mind's eye he was travelling from the Hodders on Tibbys Point to the Harbins in Rogers Cove and all the nooks and crannies in between.

As I said before Mr. Hopkins was the Lay reader in church, superintendent of Sunday school, the man behind all the happenings in Victoria Cove, the man passing out the Cocoa Malt and the Cod Liver Oil as well as making sure we got aboard the MV Christmas Seal for our checkups and X-Rays for TB. He was the man who organised the school picnics and started the three legged race and all the other fun games us

49

children took part in. He was the man who cheered when he passed out the third place ribbon as much as he cheered when he passed out the first place one. He was also the man who gave you a hearty pat on the back for trying no matter what position you came in at. He was a man of integrity; full of goodness for all mankind. He was a spiritual, confident man who knew where he was going and paved the way for many others. If I had the opportunity when I became an adult to sit and talk with him I would have told him how much he helped me especially in grade nine when I struggled with math. If there was any way for him to put an imprint inside my head he would have I'm sure.

Yes I have many memories of the man we all called Mr. Hopkins. These are but a few and I want him to know that I did fine by his teachings and still feel honoured for him to have taught me. God Bless you.

To the world you may be just one person but to one person you may be the world. author unknown

BOAT BUILDING;
GRANDFATHERS LEGACY

As a young boy growing up in Clarkes Head, Gander Bay Laurence watched his grandfather, the late Richard Gillingham build boats and knew that someday he would do the same.

By age twenty-two Laurence was married and had started a family. In the next few years he became an accomplished heavy equipment operator, working all over the Island of Newfoundland as well as on the Labrador at Churchill Falls.

That way of life was hard on the family so in nineteen seventy nine with employment only seasonal Laurence convinced himself, his wife and his children that it was better to seek full-time employment elsewhere. At that time Fort McMurray, Alberta was the choice place to be so with tears in his eyes, a few dollars in his pocket and faith for the future he pulled away from his heartbroken family for the three thousand mile journey that began with one mile at a time. That was in September and by October he had a full time job with Syncrude Canada and his family was by his side. Laurence never looked back.

With the support of his family and the seven days off that went with the Syncrude schedule Laurence started boat building. His dream was finally beginning to come true. The first two boats that he built were of ribs and planks. He cut all the timbers himself and, sawed and carved them to the shape that he needed. Those two boats were comparable to the boats that his grandfather built back in nineteen twenty nine. Yes he felt good about those boats but the climate and temperatures didn't agree with the timbers and they weren't standing up.

Laurence didn't want to give up because this was his avocation and his dream. For the next boat he decided to use cedar strip and fibreglass.

He then built a heated extension on his garage so he could work in the winter and keep his fibreglass warm and began again.

The accessibility and beauty of the rivers around Fort McMurray gave him the inspiration that he needed to pick up where his grandfather left off. Laurence still spent time with his family; we went on vacations every year and he spent hours at the Arena watching Hockey games with his son. But every spare minute was spent building boats.

Laurence was now using skill saws, jigsaws, routers and band saws and when more modern things came on the market he got them as well. He spent many moments wondering how his grandfather did it with only hand tools and the small shed he had to work in. He admired him more and more after every piece of wood he sawed. Although Laurence had upgraded from the hand tools that his grandfather used he still used some of his ideas and sometimes felt that he could hear him say, "That's right son." Sometimes things didn't go as planned but he never gave up until he got it right.

The Clearwater was the river that Laurence and his family and friends enjoyed the most. There were many Jet boats scouting up and down that river but Laurence preferred his river boat with the 15 horsepower motor. His boats had a shallow draft and could navigate in water where the jet boats dared not go. It was a far less expensive alternative to the jet set and the moderate speed allowed him to better enjoy the beauty of the river.

During those years Laurence constructed eight river boats plus a cedar strip canoe which he gave to his son and family. He took many friends and relatives on the river for day excursions and some overnight. The grandchildren enjoyed the freedom and loved to play on the sandbars. His wife Margaret enjoyed her times on the river as well. However, Margaret wanted comfort so Laurence put foam and pillows in the bottom of the boat, at the front, where she comfortably sat with her knitting and writing. Some of the poems that she has published were composed in the front of his boats or on the banks of the river with the moon shining and a campfire burning.

Laurence retired from Syncrude in December of two thousand but that didn't mean he retired from boat building. When he retired we moved to forty acres south of Athabasca which gave him lots of room and a bit more time or so he thought. With the love of any kind of wood in his veins he found himself building cupboards, cabinets, wishing wells, picnic tables, glider swings, as well as a tree house and slides for the grandchildren. He sometimes thought, "If Grandfather could see me now, what would he think? Surely he would wonder at all the fancy tools that I use. I'd like to think that I'd get a big smile from him and a pat on the back as he'd wander off to his little shed in the back."

In April of two thousand and eight along any highway from Athabasca, Alberta to Appleton, Newfoundland if you were looking in the right place you would see Laurence in a twenty four foot box cube van with his twenty five foot cedar strip boat in tow. Sixty one feet in all of precious goods that were admired at every stop he made.

Laurence's dreams have come full circle from when he was a little boy going in and out the river with his dad and his Grandfather and dreaming that one day he would have a boat of his own and as the saying goes paddle his own canoe in and out the great Gander River. Laurence lives within two minutes of the Gander River now and cherishes every moment that he spends on the river. His little boy dream of building boats that started with watching his Grandfather many years ago, has become a reality. The circle was completed when he came back home and began navigating in and out the Gander River like his Grandfather used to do. Thank you from the bottom of my heart. REST IN PEACE.

Give to the world the best you have and the best will come back to you. Author unknown

GOD BLESS ME DAD

I have many good memories of my Dad and many a story to tell. In this sitting I will try and get a couple written. My siblings and I were brought up to know right from wrong and the one thing that we learned early in life was that it was right to go to church, and wrong not to go. Now that didn't mean once a day like it is now. It meant morning service at eleven a.m., home for dinner and back to Sunday school by two p.m. Rush home again yea and you had better not loiter and play with your friends or you would be late for supper because by seven p.m. we would have to be back at the church again singing praises to the Lord. I remember that there weren't many excuses that we could have for not going to church. Maybe if we were burning up with fever or a swollen neck on both sides from the mumps we would be allowed to stay home. I'm sure it wasn't that bad but you do get my drift.

The first story that I want to tell you happened on an Easter Sunday. Dad was usually the one who walked to church with us; Mom stayed at home especially if there was a baby sibling to nurse. On this particular Easter Sunday morning dad and at least three or four siblings left the house before the sun came up because service would begin at six am. Anyone who knew Dad would know that he wasn't going to be late for anything especially the church service.

As we strolled along the outside road as we called it, we were chatting away about different things when Dad said, "I want you all to watch closely now when the sun breaks the horizon." We all questioned him but all he would say was, "You just watch now and then you'll see." Ok on we walked and talked as we strolled along the bumpy road. All of a sudden Dad said, "Look children the sun just broke the horizon and it's dancing." We looked and sure enough the sun was dancing right before our eyes. Dad told us that it was a symbol to show us that Jesus Christ had risen from the dead and the sun was dancing and rejoicing and it was a special day for us to remember. In amazement we watched as the sun continued to dance as it rose higher and higher in the sky. Was this like the Tooth Fairy, or the Easter Bunny? My young mind didn't have the answers but I put my belief in my Dad. Then in his wisdom he explained what was happening. Each step we took on the uneven ground made it look like the sun was dancing. To me it was a divine moment that has lasted through time.

Many Easter Sunday mornings as I walked with Mom and Dad and my siblings and saw the sun dance I knew in my mind that it was from our steps on the bumpy road. However, the lesson that I learned from my Dad on that special Easter Sunday morning stayed with me through the years and yes, in my heart, the sun really danced for joy just for me on those special mornings. I also learned that this was not like the Tooth Fairy at all. The sun only appeared to be dancing but for real Jesus Christ did rise from the dead on that special Easter Sunday morning many years ago. He is alive and here with us today as I still sing praises to his name.

Another Easter Sunday morning comes to mind as I reminisce about my Dad. Easter Sunday was one of the special times for the ladies of the congregation to purchase a new coat, hat, or bonnet. This particular year a new color was in and that color was Green. Needless to say most of the women were wearing some shade of green on Easter Sunday. After reciting the Canticle which began with O all ye works of the Lord bless ye the Lord, praise him and magnify him forever. And again O ye mountains and hills bless ye the Lord, praise him and magnify him forever. Well my Dad had a great sense of humour and was known to make a few people laugh in his day. This particular Easter Sunday morning was no exception. After the service, Dad with his quick step passed the ladies in the church lane and with his ready wit quoted one of the canticles loud and clear, "O all ye green things upon the earth bless ye the Lord, praise him and magnify him forever." Laughter rang out in that church lane as Dad smiled and wished everyone a Happy Easter Day. Dad has been gone now for forty four years and like another part of the Canticle says "O ye stars of heaven bless ye the Lord, praise him and magnify him forever."

Another one of my favourite memories is of spring time when the sheep gave birth to little lambs. He would come in the house all smiles and hurry us to get ready and come and see the new born lambs before we went to school. It always was a very special time to watch them

Margaret E. Peckford

grow and then one day when we'd get home from school they would be prancing around the garden and come to meet us at the gate. I still think of the lessons Dad taught me and know that he's one of those stars in heaven. GOD BLESS ME DAD

Life is like a mirror if you smile at it, it will return to you. Author unknown.

THAT'S MY MOM

I have in my treasures a few things that Mom had jotted down through the years. Sometimes it was her writings and sometimes things that she thought worthwhile to herself and others. The following verse is one of those treasures that I have had around for years. This is not only a beautiful verse; it is how my Mom looked at people and life in general.

This New Day

This brand new day is mine to spend exactly as I choose
To mark with real accomplishment or squander or misuse
To fill with love and cheerfulness or bitterness or pain
It is my choice to make this day a total loss or gain
So counsel and direct me Lord that when this day shall end
I may rejoice with work well done be richer by a friend
And when I sleep may angels pause beside your throne and tell
That I have lived this day of mine not wastefully but well.

My Mom's journey on this earth ended when she was only sixty-seven years old; a short journey but one filled to the brim with love and inspiration that she passed on to others. Her earthly journey is still continuing in the hearts and minds of all those who loved her. When it comes to a long life span it didn't seem to happen with my parents because my Dad died at age sixty-one. Mom was age forty-nine when Dad died and she was left to raise an eight year old son and a teenage daughter. It was never easy and often a struggle to make ends meet.

Mom was never what you would call a healthy woman. I remember from an early age how arthritis crippled her whole body. When I would come home from school I would see her pushing a chair in front of her for support to get to the oven to check on supper, the homemade bread or to put a few junks of wood in the stove. But when I would ask her how she was feeling she would always say, "Not so bad today my dear I can get around a bit better today." Mom never complained or I didn't hear any of it. Sometimes she would lie on the daybed and she would say, "For a ten minute cat nap and that will get me through until bedtime. That's my Mom.

At our home there was always something to do and that meant for everyone. Mom always said, "This is for your own good because someday when the time comes for you to be on your own you will know how to clean and cook." She also taught us that anything worth doing was worth doing well. God bless her heart. I have thanked her many times through the years although at the time it was hard to have to do the jobs before we could go and play. They were jobs then not chores like it is today. Each of us would have our jobs to do especially on Saturday. We would start upstairs making beds and cleaning and dusting until we completed the four rooms, the upper hall, the stair head and the fifteen steps to the hall below. You talk about a place getting scrubbed; every table, every chair and chair rung had to be cleaned, all the shoes taken out from under the daybed and everything cleaned and the shoes put back in order.

Mom could turn her hand to most anything. With all of us young ones there was always clothes to wash, which was mostly done on Mondays. I remember in the summer when school was closing it would be announced in church and school that the church would be cleaned the first fine day after Monday. Everyone knew that wash day was Monday and from one end of Victoria Cove to the other every clothes line would be full. Mom scrubbed our clothes on the wash board in the early years. Later she had a gas wringer washer that was hard to start and made a loud noise. Clothes would get caught in the wringer just when she thought she was making headway. She always tried to get the clothes on the line early morning especially in the winter to catch the little sun that we got. Of course in the winter clothes still froze on the line in full form. In the spring when the weather was good the un-mentionable would happen; the clothes line would break and the whole shebang would be down in the mud. Sometimes the horses would walk under the clothes and mess them up. Mom had lots of patience, bless her heart; the only thing to do was bring it all in and do it over again. That's my Mom.

Mom sewed and mended some days from morning until night. She made most of our clothes. I remember her taking one of her coats that she had worn for years and rip it all apart, turn it inside out, cut out a pattern and make a coat for one of the girls that looked brand new. Mom could also knit like the trooper as they say. We would lose a mitt at school and by morning there would be another one ready for us. I specially remember Mom knitting the Mary Maxim sweaters when they were popular. We all had to have one and all with different patterns. At that time our youngest brother Lorne was small and got into all kinds of mischief. He would pull the needles out of a sweater that she was knitting, usually at the most difficult part of the pattern. But Mom persevered and knit three or four sweaters that winter. I can see her now sitting on the edge of the table so that Lorne couldn't reach her needles. What a woman! That's my Mom.

For years Mom made and baked bread and cooked meals every day as well as looking after all the other needs of us children. Grandfather and Grandmother King lived with us and she looked after the both of them until they went to their eternal rest. With eight of us to care for I wonder how many snotty noses she wiped? How many scraped knees and elbows she attended to? How many sleepless nights she had when we all had our childhood diseases? When we had the whooping cough she'd spend the night walking the floor with one of us in her arms or on her knees praying for daylight to come and to know that we had made it through another night. There were no doctors to take care of us so she had to make use of all the home remedies that she knew of. She would burn flour for diaper rash; use hot water bottles to relieve an ear ache, tooth ache or tummy ache; heat a brick on the stove and wrap it in cloths and put in your bed to help keep your feet warm; she would place a towel over the sick child's head and a pan or kettle of boiling water and use the steam to relieve the croup; use Vicks VapoRub on the chest, covered with red flannel to relieve a cough or cold and burn sulphur on the stove to help prevent others from catching whatever disease that was in the home.

Our home was a place where everyone gathered. Our cousins and friends came from near and far to swim in the summer and our pathway had the deepest groves from playing hop-scotch. Mom was a good listener and our friends came to her and talked about their little puppy love issues. Mom also had a good shoulder to cry on and I came to her lots of times when someone hurt me at school. Yes my Mom was a gentle soul, who spent many long hours making things right for her family.

We would all sit around the kitchen table and do our reading, writing and arithmetic in the glow of the kerosene lamp. We also learned our Sunday school lesson, collects, creeds and Catechism. Mom taught us our prayers; "Now I lay me down to sleep etc." We were happy when there was time left over to learn how to play cribbage and one hundreds and twenties. I also loved to play my IQ game to try and beat Mom and Dad.

Mom had a strong faith and believed in prayer. Many times I would hear her say, "My dear more things are wrought by prayer than this world dreams off." Two of her favourite passages in the Bible were John's Gospel chapter 14 where it says, "In my father's house there are many mansions; I go to prepare a place for you." She also found comfort in the verses of the twenty-third psalm.

I was talking to Mrs. Irene Webb the other day and she told me how blessed that she was to know my Mom. Mrs. Webb was superintendent of the Sunday school for many years and used to visit mom on her way back from school. This of course was after Mom lost the old family home and everything in it by fire and she lived down around the cove as we called it in John and Beulah's little house. Mrs. Webb told me she learned so much from Mom. Even with losing everything she was always so thankful for what she had. Mom suffered for years with arthritis but very seldom was there a complaint. Her lungs were also real bad and her cough was deep and irritating. Even with all her physical problems she always had a smile and a kind word and was always more concerned with how you were doing. Mom never said anything bad about anyone and she always taught us children that if we couldn't say anything good about anyone it was better not to say anything at all.

Mom was the Tooth Fairy, Santa Claus, Easter Bunny, Nurse, Doctor, Barber, Tailor, Cook, Housekeeper, Teacher, and the best friend in the world. She could churn butter, milk cows, set and dig potatoes, look after hens and sheep and lend a hand to an aunt across the road if need be. Back in those early days most Moms and Dads didn't say I love you like they do today. Their actions spoke louder than words and some-how we knew that when we got tucked in at night, found a warm brick in our bed and blankets that weighed heavy on us to keep us warm when the easterly winds beat in on the shore, yes we knew we were loved a whole bunch.

I can hear Mom singing, "Take my life and let it be consecrated Lord to thee." Mom made us a family with her inner strength. She made our house a home with her love and faith. She has made her home in Heaven and is safe in the arms of Jesus.

That's my Mom. God bless her.

Love is missing someone whenever you're apart, but somehow feeling warm inside because you're close in heart. Author unknown.

THE BEST DOG EVER

By Kailey Peckford

Loyal, friendly, brave;
that's the dog I knew and loved;
Watching over me.

We grew together;
He would never leave my side;
He was so gentle.

He was a big dog;
So strong and mighty, but
He grew very old.

His legs they failed him
but he was alive at the heart
Taz, we miss you so.

If there is a doggy heaven
I know that's where you are
we'll always remember you Taz.

In Remembrance of Taz because he truly was the best
Dog ever
P.S. Say Hi to Smokey for me

103-26 153rd. Street
Edmonton, Alberta
T5P 2B8

THE OWL AND I

The first sentences that I can remember putting together was the prayer that I said by Mom or Dads knee and it was, "In my little bed I lie, Heavenly father hear my cry, Lord protect me through the night and keep me safe till morning light." Then I probably learnt the verses "Roses are Red Violets are Blue Sugar is Sweet and so are you." In first grade or Primer as it was called then I read about Dick, Jane, Sally, Spot and of course Puff the kitten.

I vividly remember learning the famous poem "The Owl and the Pussy Cat" which I know now was written by Edward Lear the English painter and humorist. He was also considered to be among the greatest masters of the witty, light verse known as the limerick. Also at a very early age my Dad taught me this verse about an Owl. "The wise old Owl sat on an oak; the more he saw the less he spoke; the less he spoke the more he heard; why can't we all be like that old bird?" Many times through my life I have reflected on that verse and the lessons one could learn by following that great old bird.

When I went in the woods with Dad on the bob sleds to haul out the long turns of fire wood sometime during the winter season we would spy an Owl sitting in a tree along the wood road. We would see other animals and birds as well but the Owl always caught my attention the most. When I was eight years old and had to spend time in the hospital at Twillingate, before Mom went home she brought me some goodies one of which was the book "The Owl and the Pussy Cat." I loved that book with all my heart; it was a fairly large book with only a few pages. The material in the cover was cloth with a little shine to it. The colors were beautiful and the words soothing to me at a time when I needed it.

When I was growing up I was in both the Brownies and Girl Guides. One of our leaders in Brownies was Mrs. Mildred Torraville who was Tawnie Owl. We had so much fun and did lots of different activities at our meetings and special entertainment days. On one occasion we had a talent and costume show. I wanted to go dressed as an owl and my Mom, bless her heart made a special owl costume for me. I flew across the stage and perched on a piece of wood and quoted the poem about the wise old owl that Dad had taught me. To the delight of both Mom and myself I won the prize for the best and funniest costume, again making the Owl a significant part of my life.

Through the years I did quite a bit of reading and sometimes I would just open a book at random and there would be something there about the owl. One of those books is the Holy Bible where the owl is mentioned in the book of Leviticus, the book of Psalms and the book of Isaiah.

During almost thirty years in Alberta we did quite a bit of traveling. On one of our trips we stopped in at the Alberta Bird Sanctuary. It was an amazing place and again I was drawn to the Owl and needless to say I had my picture taken with the Owl sitting on my fingers. Of course I told him how very wise he was and he rotated his head for me as if to say thank you. I also told him the story my Dad told me long ago and how proud I was that he was perched on my fingers as if he didn't have a care in the world, how wise.

One day in the early nineties I was at the home of my friend the Rev. Jody Miles helping her sort out her office. One of the tasks that she asked me to do was sort through her library and arrange her books. As I stood looking at the six or seven rows of books that covered one wall of the office I gasped as my eye caught the name of the book, "I Heard the Owl Call My Name." Wow! I was about to learn another lesson in life. I told my friend a few things about the owl in my life and I was about to borrow the book from her when we found the second book so she gave me one to keep. It is a story of life, love, courage and dignity of one man's truths of human existence. Even now when I look at my small library my eyes will focus on the little book tucked in among the bigger ones. Something draws me to this book and I often take it out and read a few paragraphs from it.

Through the years I have looked everywhere for the book 'The Owl and The Pussy Cat."I I even wrote to the publisher of Golden Books at one time but wasn't successful in getting one. I was helping to organize a selection of books at a church office a few years back and I spotted a couple of small books. I told them some of my story and was gracefully given the books. A few years ago when I opened a birthday gift from my oldest daughter Angela I found elegantly printed on card paper the story of "The Owl and The Pussy Cat." My eyes filled with tears just to know that she knew it would mean a lot to me. Thank you so much sweetie.

Also on my life's journey I have had to seek professional help from time to time and one of the Places that my Doctor referred me to was none other than "White Owl Mind and Body Work." How the universe works amazes me no end.

I feel in my heart that the Owl has represented leadership in my life. Leadership provided by my Dad, Mom, Brownie and Girl Guide leaders as well as comfort to me when I felt all alone at the hospital. Leadership provided by the Rev. Jody Miles and the book she gave me when I volunteered my services and comfort from the Holy Bible; the word of God.

Still today as I travel from place to place I keep a watchful eye on the birds of prey and I know somewhere waiting to teach me another lesson is that Wise Old Owl.

It's not what happens to us but how we react to what happens to us. Author unknown

THE SEAT BROKE IN LITTLE PIECES

I was eight years old and it was my first time in Hospital. That in itself was a disturbing time for me. In telling about my time in the Hospital I will also tell you of the experience we had in getting to and from Twillingate Hospital during November and December month in nineteen fifty-two. Mom and Dad knew something was wrong with me after I slowly made it home from school a bit late one Friday afternoon. I was in pain and bent over because my stomach was so tender and I could hardly walk. Mom and Dad knew what had to be done but at that time of year it was going to be risky. They made me as comfortable as possible and made arrangements to go to Twillingate on Monday.

Uncle Louis Porter ran a passenger boat at the time and had made many trips in rough waters. He also had more passengers on board that Monday morning my Uncle Lloyd and my cousin Eric were travelling with us. Eric was also sick with a bad stomach much the same as myself. The trip up there was a bit bumpy to say the least but after a few hours we made it to the Island. A taxi took us to the Hospital and we got to see the Doctor. Old Doctor Olds was there at that time and took one look at us and pushed on our bellies and right away he said Appendicitis and we were admitted immediately. Emergency surgery scheduled for both of us.

Mom and Uncle Lloyd had to leave right away but not before she brought me a couple of treats and a story book. It was the big one with sort of oilcloth covering on it and the title was The Owl and the Pussy Cat. I cried to break my heart when Mom left to go home that day but I knew she had to go because there was a big family still at home to care for. I treasured that book and read it every day when I began to feel better. I will never forget the smell of ether that they used to put me to sleep.

They put this cloth over my mouth and nose and asked me to breath in and out it was awful I felt like they were smothering me and I cried for Mom to come and get me. Then of course I knew nothing until I was wrenching my guts out from the after effects of the ether and surgery. But after a few days I was feeling better and was out of bed running around waiting for Mom to come and get me.

Eric on the other hand wasn't as lucky as I was; by the time they did his surgery his appendix had ruptured. He was a sick five year old boy for a long time. He was on the same ward as I was but he was in a crib and I was in a regular hospital bed. I could see him and hear him cry for his Mummy and Daddy and that didn't help me none. I spent a lot of time crying the days turned into a week and on and on. I was feeling good so why couldn't I go home. Why wasn't Mom or Dad here to get me? I learned after that Eric had to stay a month because his appendix ruptured and I had to stay too because they couldn't make two trips to Twillingate to get us that time of the year. On Sundays the children would come by the windows and show us their Sunday school papers and during the week their school work. That was fun and kept us company for a little while but the time was long and if Dr. Olds caught us in the hallways you could hear him grumble to get back in your bed although he was a very nice man could get "gruffy" sometimes. The nurses were sweet and let us help them sometimes.

Then one day while I was sitting up in bed with my arms around my knees rocking back and forth back and forth I heard my name and when I looked up my Mom was standing in the doorway with Uncle Lloyd close behind. I ran to her and we hugged and hugged and I was still crying but they were tears of joy this time.

Now this was supposed to be the good part but it was a nightmare instead. It was now the eighteenth of December my sister Enid's birthday and a stormy day it was. Uncle Louis wouldn't take a chance to come around the cape so we had to take a smaller boat to cross some water to get to his bigger boat which wasn't supposed to be so bad. We all piled into this little motor boat and left the land behind. Within five minutes we were in open water and the little boat was tossing up and down on the waves. I was holding on to Mom who was holding on to a helpful man from Summerside and Uncle Lloyd had Eric in his arms. Eric was crying Daddy we are going to drown and I was crying and holding on for dare life when we heard a shout from above us and a man said sorry we have to close the hatch door. Now we were in the dark and the wind was stronger and the waves higher. Now we were banging up and now on the waves. I heard something cracking and screamed but the man from Summerford in a soft spoken voice said don't worry about that it's only the seat splitting beneath us. Now some of us were on the floor and holding each other real tight in the cuddy of the boat. It seemed like forever and then we were in the calm waters. Everyone was thanking God for their safety. Even with all this fear and I was only eight years old I was remembering the story of Jesus and his disciples on the Sea of Galilee. It was really my first test of faith in Jesus. In my eight year old mind I asked Jesus to keep us safe and calm the sea as He calmed the raging sea for his disciples. When I told my mom she just smiled and said yes my dear a little child shall lead them.

By the time we landed on the dock the sky was clouded over and it was getting dark and our journey wasn't over yet. We still had a hard walk ahead of us. So with Uncle Louis with his lantern to guide us we made our way across railway ties. Uncle Lloyd carried Eric but I was too heavy for Mom and our steps were so short we had to take two steps to get across the ties. This was just some of the hardships that were faced back in the fifties and especially during the winter time. Everyone took it in stride; sometimes there was loss of lives because of the travelling conditions but for us I guess you could call it a bump in the waves. Sometime later that night we made it to Uncle Louis's boat and continued on our journey home. The excitement at our home was three fold because I was home after being away for a month and Mom was home again and there were candles to be blown out by Enid, Happy Birthday to be sung and delicious chocolate cake to be enjoyed by all. I was so happy I thought I would burst; I was home again safe warm and Christmas Day was next week.

The storms are needed to point out how well we're prepared. Author unknown.

A CERTAIN MOMENT
Author Unknown

At a certain moment a doctor will determine that my brain has ceased to function and that, for all intents and purposes, my life has stopped. When that happens, do not attempt to instil artificial life into my body by the use of a machine. And do not call this my death bed. Call it my, Bed of life, and let my body be taken from it to help others lead fuller lives.

Give my sight to a man who has never seen a sunrise, a baby's face or love in the eyes of a woman. Give my heart to a person whose heart has caused nothing but endless days of pain. Give my blood to the teenager who has been pulled from the wreckage of his car, so that he might live to see his grandchildren play. Give my kidneys to one who depends on a machine to exist from week to week. Take my bones, every muscle, every fibre and nerve in my body and find a way to make a crippled child walk. Explore every corner of my brain. Take my cells, if necessary, and let them grow so that someday a speechless boy will shout at the crack of a bat and a deaf girl will hear the sound of rain against her window. Burn what is left of me and scatter my ashes to the winds to help the flowers grow. If you must bury something, let it be my faults, my weaknesses and all unkind thoughts against my fellow man. Give my soul to God. If by chance you wish to remember me, do it with a kind deed or word to someone who needs you. If you do all I ask, I will live forever.

These words were such an inspiration to me and so much the way I feel that I wanted to share them with all of you.

WHY WOMEN CRY

A little boy asked his mother, "Why are you crying?"
"Because I am a woman," she told him. "I don't understand," he said.
His mom just hugged him and said, "And you never will.'
Later the little boy asked his father, "Why does mother seem to cry for
no reason?"
"All women cry for no reason," was all his dad could say.
The little boy grew up and became a man, still wondering why women
cry.
Finally he put in a call to God.
When God got on the phone he asked, "God, why do women cry so
easily?"
God said, "When I made the woman she had to be special. I made her
shoulders strong enough to carry the weight of the world, yet gentle
enough to give comfort.
I gave her an inner strength to endure childbirth and the reject on that
many times comes from her children.
I gave her a hardness that allows her to keep going when everyone
else gives up and take care of her family through sickness and fatigue
without complaining.
I gave her the sensitivity to love her children under all circumstances
even when her child has hurt her badly.
I gave her strength to carry her husband through his faults and
fashioned her from his rib to protect his heart.
I gave her wisdom to know that a good husband never hurts his wife
but sometimes tests her strengths and her resolve to stand by him
unfailingly.
And finally gave her a tear to shed. This is hers exclusively to use
whenever it is needed.
"You see my son," said God, "The beauty of a woman is not in the
clothes she wears, the figure that she carries, or the way she combs her
hair.
The beauty of a woman must be seen in her eyes, because that is the
doorway to her heart, the place where love resides. Author unknown.

OUR YELLOW, FLARED-TAIL DRESSES

We were going to be the belle of the ball or in this case the belle of the garden party.

Mom had spent hours sewing our beautiful, bright, sunshine yellow flared-tail dresses for us to debut at the garden party. The dresses had black sashes around the waist and we wore a black bow in our hair. To top off the attire we wore pop-corn bobby socks with laced up black shoes. We were going to look spiffy thanks to Mom. We probably dreamed about this party for weeks now, but some dreams are short lived and this was to be one of them

Mom was away in Grand Falls getting dentures; probably her first ones. At that time Grand Falls seemed far away but that is where she had to go and she had to stay a few days. Dad was looking after us, while the older girls were helping with our younger brother Mark and baby sister Enid. Well she wasn't really a baby; she was four years old. But at that time she was the baby of the family and spoiled rotten I might add

The August morning of the garden party dawned sunny and bright and our spirits were high. In fact not much else was on our minds as we hurriedly did our jobs so we could don our new dresses and be at the school grounds on time. In the meantime Dad was in the potato garden and Enid was playing with her little boat in a ditch with a little muddy water in it. We were supposed to be watching her at all times but I guess the anticipation of the afternoon of fun we about to enjoy was the uppermost thing on our minds and somehow forgot Enid for a moment. She chose that moment to fall face first into the ditch. Dad saw her about the same time we did and ran screaming toward us we pulled her out by the straps of her overhauls, Oh my God we were all so frightened but Enid just spluttered for a couple seconds and then gave us a big smile.

Now for the cleanup; the garden party and the yellow, flared-tail dresses were put in the back of our minds as we warmed water and got out the big wash tub and took off the muddy clothes and dunked her in. Her long blond naturally curly hair was a sight to see. As we washed her we laughed and cried at the same time. Supposing she had smothered in the ditch; look what Mom would have to face when she came home. Dad was already so upset with us that we were going to have to watch our p's and q's to get back in his good books.

We knew without a doubt that we wouldn't get to the garden party that afternoon. You know it didn't bother us at all as we washed her and changed waters thirteen times before we got her presentable. She just shined from all the washing and her beautiful curly hair was blond again when we took her to Dad who was waiting in the rocking chair in the kitchen. We heard a big sigh of relief from him as he took her in h s arms and hugged her. We learnt a big lesson that day and all three of us looked pretty humble when we walked to church on Sunday donning our bright yellow, flared-tail dresses. We were thankful that Mom was home and that our baby sister was just fine.

God didn t promise days without rain, laughter without sorrow or sun without rain. But God did promise strength for the day, comfort for the tears and light for the way. And for all who believe in his kingdom above he answers their faith with everlasting Love. Author unknown.

THIS CUP AND SAUCER

I gave a little cup and saucer to each of my
Grandchildren that was filled with cut decorations of all
shapes.

In this cup and saucer I'm giving you
There is a love that has no end
Hugs and kissed and sweet dreams
Filled to the very brim.

Each year as you grow older take down this little cup
Remember that each hug and kiss was from Grandma's
loving touch.

You may choose a hug, a kiss, a dream each year will be
your choice
But no matter where your Grandma is she will listen to
your sweet voice.

Each day of our lives we make deposits in the memory banks of our children. Author unknown

www.ingramcontent.com/pod-product-compliance
Lightning Source LLC
Chambersburg PA
CBHW021230280526
45784CB00005B/2036